YOU'RE CELESTIAL

GUIDE TO YOUR SHADOWS

MATTHEW TRAN

Balboa Press books may be ordered through booksellers or by contacting:

Balboa Press
A Division of Hay House
1663 Liberty Drive
Bloomington, IN 47403
www.balboapress.com
844-682-1282

ISBN: 979-8-7652-4742-6 (sc)
ISBN: 979-8-7652-4741-9 (e)

Library of Congress Control Number: 2023922008

Print information available on the last page.

Balboa Press rev. date: 08/14/2024

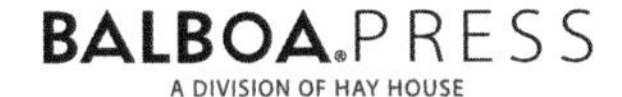

OUR LIVES

ARE NON-LINEAR.
JOURNEYS OF SELF-COMPASSION...

Exploration of one's own depths & darkness leads to and uncovers many blessings within.

ONE DAY AT A TIME.
PACE YOURSELF.

REVEAL AND RECOVER TREASURES.
RECLAIM THE PAST.

The Universe supports you! Reflect upon all the beautiful facets in you. Release and let go of what is no longer serving you. Make room for what does.

GROUND DAILY.

FIND GRATITUDE FOR CHALLENGES & BLESSINGS.

IF LOST ON ANY TOPIC, READ THE MYTHOLOGY, STORIES, OR SEEK OTHERS FOR GUIDANCE.

IF THERE ISN'T ENOUGH ROOM TO WRITE, ADD STICKY-NOTES OR PAPER. THIS AREA COULD BE AN IMPORTANT EMPHASIS WITHIN YOUR CHART.

KEY RESOURCES

& INSTRUCTIONS TO GET THE MOST OPTIMAL EXPERIENCE.

ASTRO-SEEK.COM

1. CLICK BIRTH CHART & ENTER YOUR INFORMATION.
2. CLICK EXTENDED SETTINGS.
3. CHANGE THE HOUSE SYSTEM TO WHOLE SIGN AND CHANGE TROPICAL ZODIAC TO SIDEREAL-LAHIRI.
4. CLICK CALCULATE CHART

I prefer Sidereal because It resonates more and incorporates the 26,000 year Yuga cycles.

TO FIND YOUR PERSONAL HOUSE PLACEMENTS, LOOK FOR THE SYMBOLS OF THE PLANETS. FIND THE PIE CHART WEDGE THE PLANET IS SITTING IN. NUMBERS FOR EACH WEDGE ARE THE HOUSE NUMBERS.

- **Use a search engine you are familiar with (Google, Yahoo, or anything of that nature) for each topic.**
- **Reading at least 3 different astrological websites can provide a decent perspective.**
- **Image and explanation for the 12 houses is found at astrostyle.com/astrology/12-zodiac-houses**

ADDITIONAL RESOURCES

1. ADVANCED-ASTROLOGY.COM
2. HOROSCOPE.COM
3. CAFEASTROLOGY.COM
4. ASTROLOGY.COM
5. ASTRO.COM
6. YOUTUBE - SOUL NAVIGATION ASTROLOGY & TAROT CHANNEL OR @SOULNAVIGATION

Using AI resources, like ChatGPT, can be very helpful with formulating notes, (e.g. asking ChatGPT, "What gives the Sun in the 12th house fuel?")

HOUSE PLACEMENTS & GENERALIZED DESCRIPTIONS

FILL IN THE BLANKS BELOW:

1. Sun in the ______ House • Area for vitality or life force
2. Moon in the ______ House • Area for emotional support
3. Mercury in the ______ House • Area for processing thoughts
4. Venus in the ______ House • Area of values & attraction
5. Mars in the ______ House • Area where passion flares
6. Jupiter in the ______ House • Area where you are naturally blessed
7. Saturn in the ______ House • Area of pressures or discipline
8. Uranus in the ______ House • Area that is most unconventional
9. Neptune in the ______ House • Area that feels dreamy or hazy
10. Pluto in the ______ House • Area that can feel transformative or powerful

THE SUN

VITALITY & LIFE FORCE

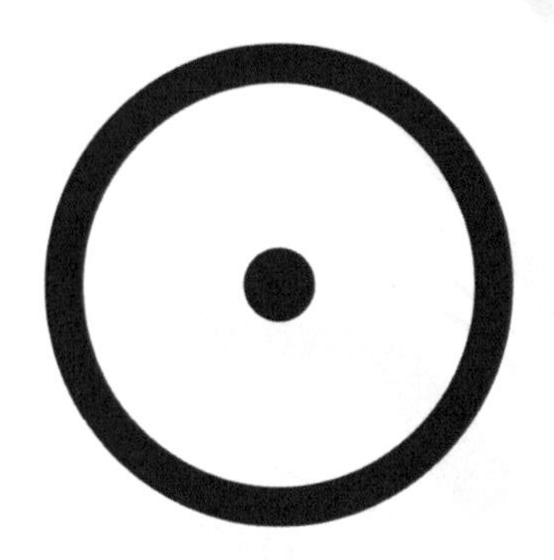

The area where you find the Sun often provides you with vitality and life force. Spending time daily with the energy of the house that has your Sun in it, is capable of recharging your batteries.

SPEND TIME IN THE ENERGY OF YOUR _____ HOUSE SUN. DAILY! WITH LOW BATTERIES, MOST PROCESSING CAN FEEL SLOW.

Reflect & Journal: HOW CAN I RECHARGE MY BATTERIES DAILY?

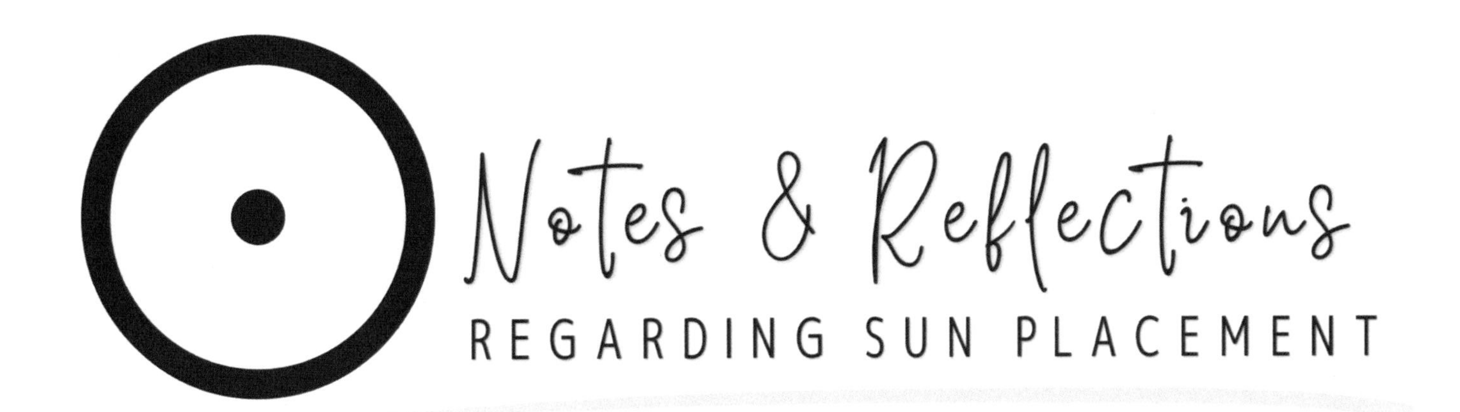
Notes & Reflections
REGARDING SUN PLACEMENT

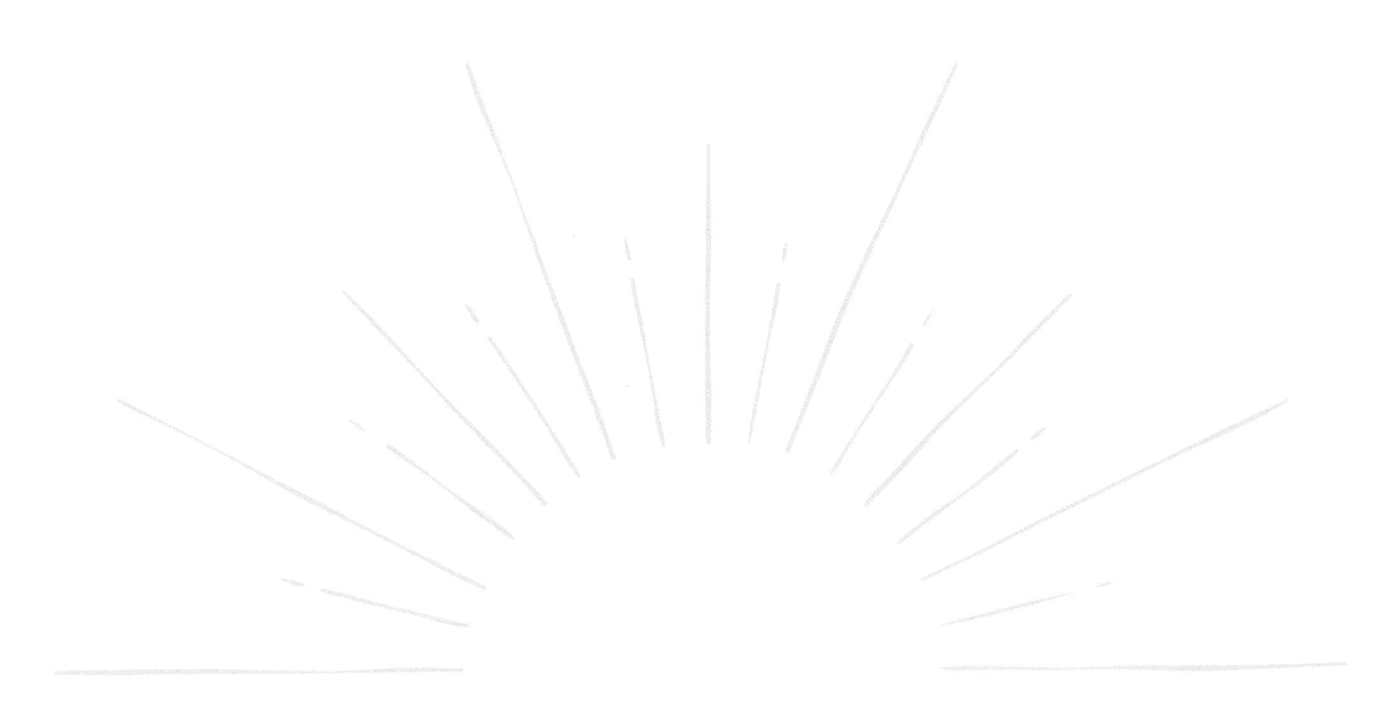

THE MOON

EMOTIONAL SUPPORT & NURTURING

Throughout the course of your journey, processing the emotions that arise can be very important.

SPENDING TIME IN THE ENERGY OF YOUR _____ HOUSE MOON CAN GIVE YOU THE EMOTIONAL SUPPORT TO HANDLE WHAT MAY SURFACE. GROUNDING IS ESSENTIAL.

Reflect & Journal: HOW CAN I ACCESS THIS ENERGY?

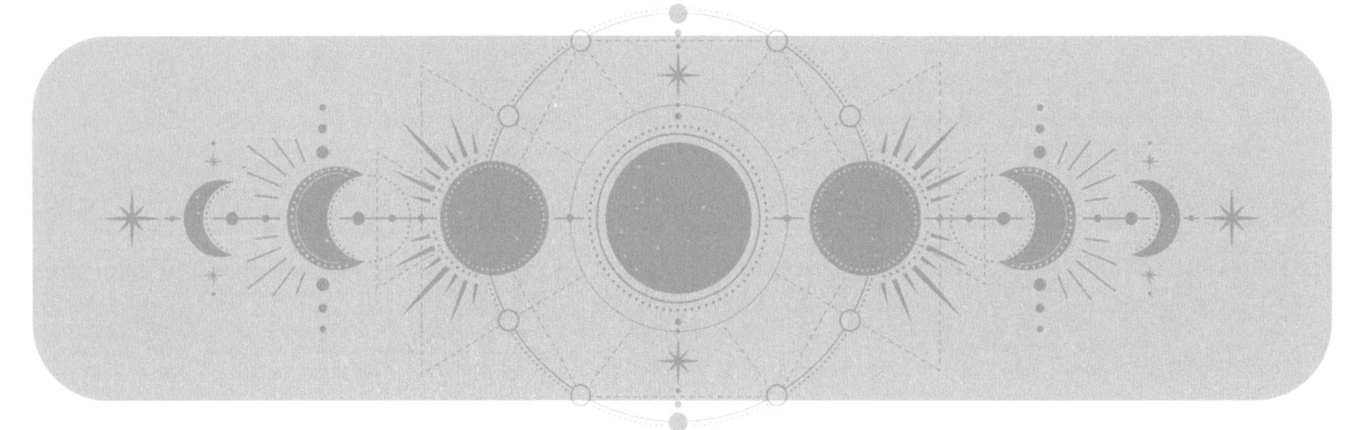

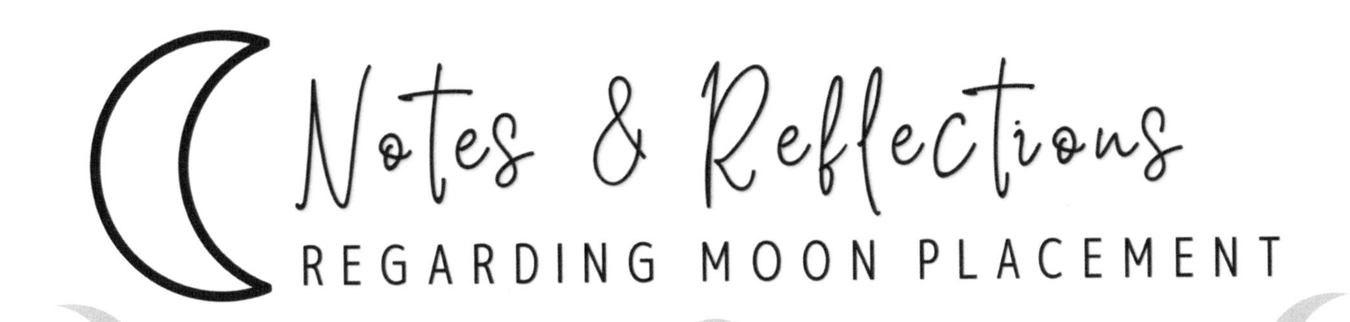

ADDITIONAL WEBSITES FOR THE MOON:

ELITEDAILY.COM - WHAT HOUSE IS YOUR MOON SIGN IN?
YOURTANGO.COM - HOW TO USE THE HOUSE YOUR MOON IS IN TO CONNECT EMOTIONS.

MERCURY

MIND & LOGIC

The house that Mercury is placed in reveals how you tend to process thoughts in the most efficient way. Highly suggested to work on and contemplate this book within the energy of your Mercury placement. If you have trouble finding an answer, go here.

MERCURY IN THE ____ HOUSE.

Reflect & Journal:

HOW CAN I ACCESS THIS ENERGY? HOW DO I MAKE THIS ACCESSIBLE THROUGHOUT THE COURSE OF THIS WORKBOOK?

ALONE? IN THE LIVING ROOM? TALKING THINGS OUT? WITH FAMILY? ON THE PATIO? COFFEE SHOP OR A LIBRARY? SURROUNDED BY COMMUNITY? WITH FRIEND?

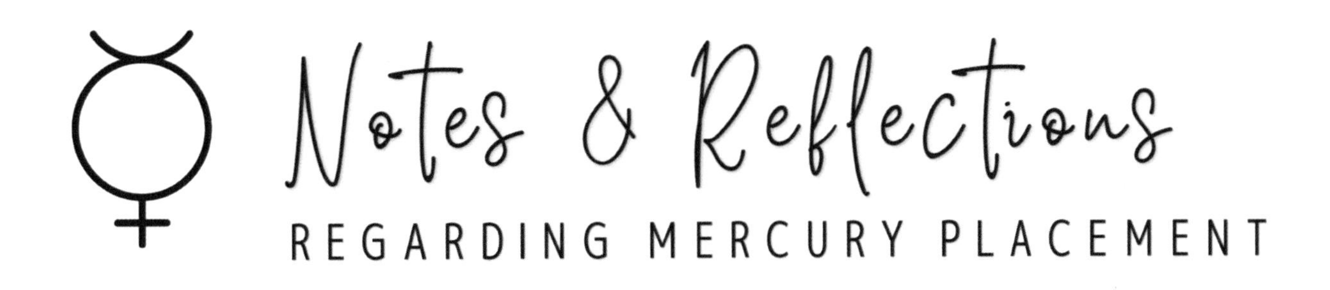
Notes & Reflections
REGARDING MERCURY PLACEMENT

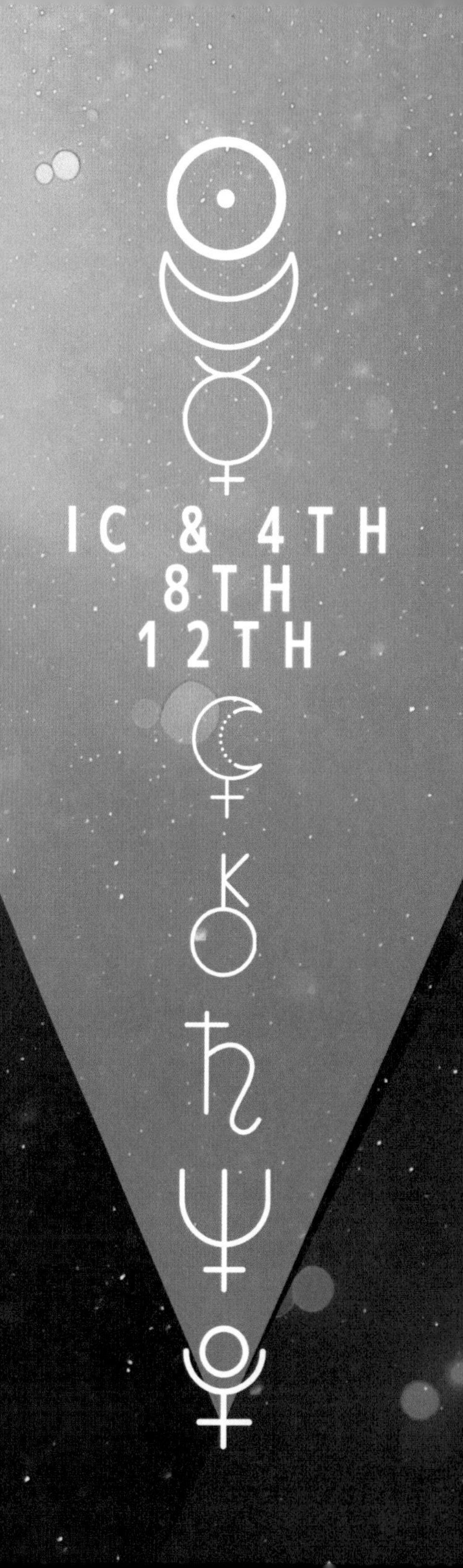
IC & 4TH
8TH
12TH

CAUTION

BE ADVISED:

BEFORE DOING ANY OF THE FOLLOWING PAGES, MAKE SURE TO USE GROUNDING METHODS AND SPEND TIME IN YOUR SUN'S HOUSE ENERGY.

MY RECOMMENDATIONS ARE AS FOLLOWS:

DO ONLY ONE PAGE A DAY.
GIVE EACH AREA THE ATTENTION, RESPECT, AND PATIENCE NEEDED FOR HEALING.

WRITE AS MUCH AS YOU CAN WITH THE SPACE AVAILABLE.
KNOWLEDGE IS KEY IN VIEWING PERSPECTIVES OF CHALLENGES AND BLESSINGS. IF YOU RUN OUT OF SPACE AND NEED TO EXPAND, ADD STICKY NOTES OR EXTRA PAGES AS NEEDED.

FOR EVERY CHALLENGE PLACED UPON US, THERE IS A BLESSING. IT IS TIME TO RETRIEVE THOSE TREASURES.

IMUM COELI | IC

INNER CHILD

IC YOUR IMUM COELI IS IN THE ____ HOUSE.

YOUR IC IS IN THE ASTROLOGICAL SIGN OF

________________________ .

Fourth House

HOUSE OF LINEAGE, SOMETIMES GHOSTS.

YOUR 4TH HOUSE ASTROLOGICAL SIGN IS:

ARE THERE ANY PLANETS LOCATED IN THIS HOUSE?

4TH HOUSE

Tread with Awareness & Without Judgement.

ALLOW FEELING, SIT IN IT, EXPRESS IT. THROUGH YOUR MOON, LET GO OF RESISTING, LET FEELINGS FLOW THROUGH TO THE SURFACE, TO THE LIGHT.

WRITE & EXPRESS THESE FEELINGS. REPEAT THIS PART AS NEEDED FOR DEEP EMOTIONS TO SETTLE.

4TH HOUSE

TRANSMUTE, INTEGRATE, & RENOVATE:

Challenges and Blessings

CHALLENGES FOUND THROUGH RESEARCH	BLESSINGS FOUND THROUGH RESEARCH

MY OWN LIFE EXAMPLES OF THESE CHALLENGES:

MY OWN LIFE EXPERIENCES OF THESE BLESSINGS:

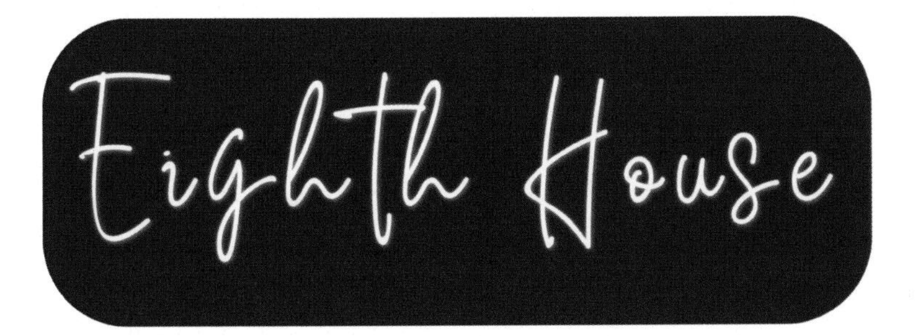

HOUSE OF INTIMACY, SOMETIMES DEMONS

YOUR 8TH HOUSE ASTROLOGICAL SIGN IS:

ARE THERE ANY PLANETS LOCATED IN THIS HOUSE?

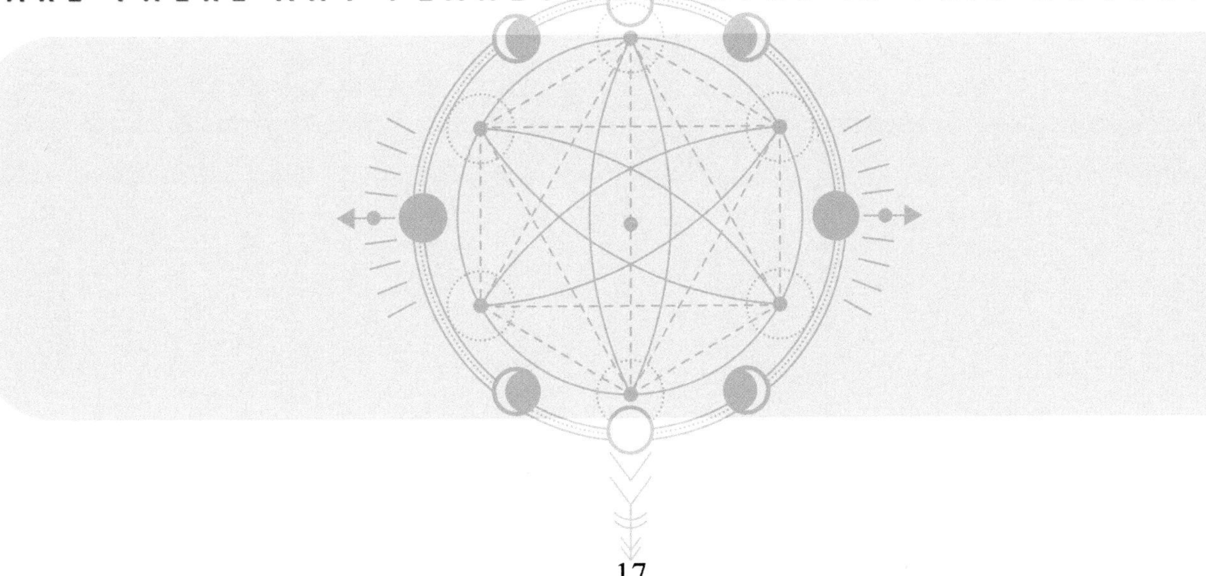

8TH HOUSE

Tread with Awareness & Without Judgement.

ALLOW FEELING, SIT IN IT, EXPRESS IT. THROUGH YOUR MOON, LET GO OF RESISTING, LET FEELINGS FLOW THROUGH TO THE SURFACE, TO THE LIGHT.

WRITE & EXPRESS THESE FEELINGS. REPEAT THIS PART AS NEEDED FOR DEEP EMOTIONS TO SETTLE.

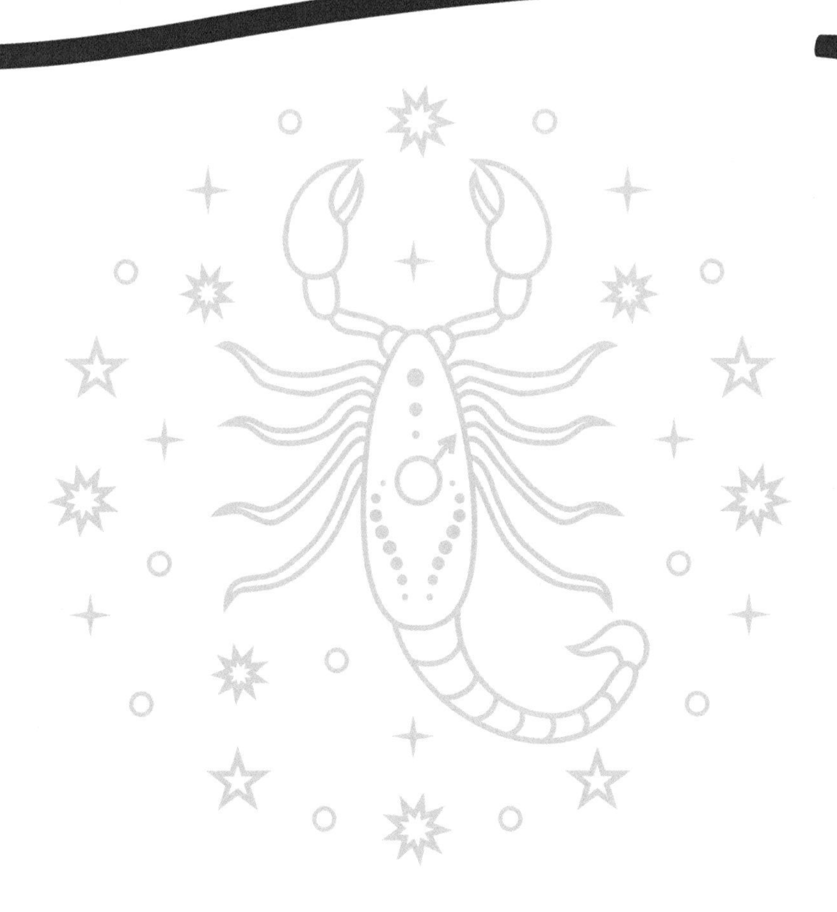

8TH HOUSE
TRANSMUTE, INTEGRATE, & RENOVATE:
Challenges and Blessings

CHALLENGES FOUND THROUGH RESEARCH	BLESSINGS FOUND THROUGH RESEARCH

MY OWN LIFE EXAMPLES OF THESE CHALLENGES:

MY OWN LIFE EXPERIENCES OF THESE BLESSINGS:

Twelfth House

HOUSE OF DREAMS, SOMETIMES NIGHTMARES.

YOUR 12TH HOUSE ASTROLOGICAL SIGN IS:

ARE THERE ANY PLANETS LOCATED IN THIS HOUSE?

12TH HOUSE

Tread with Awareness & Without Judgement.

ALLOW FEELING, SIT IN IT, EXPRESS IT. THROUGH YOUR MOON, LET GO OF RESISTING, LET FEELINGS FLOW THROUGH TO THE SURFACE, TO THE LIGHT.

WRITE & EXPRESS THESE FEELINGS. REPEAT THIS PART AS NEEDED FOR DEEP EMOTIONS TO SETTLE.

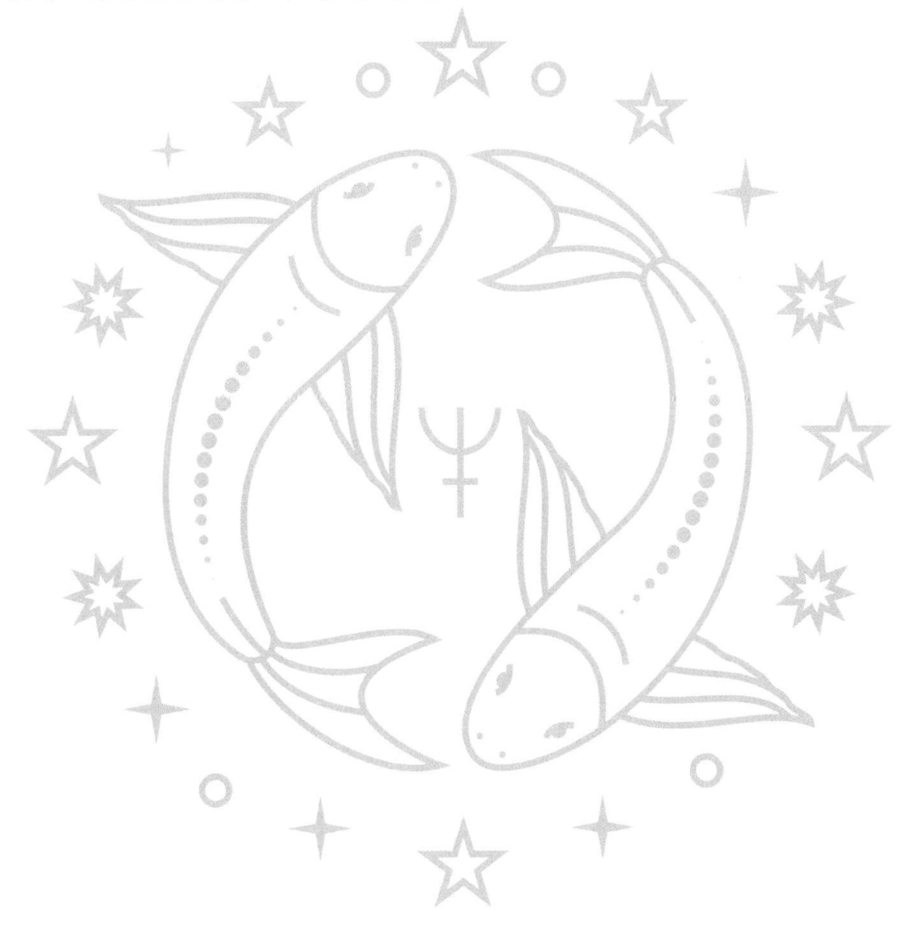

12TH HOUSE
TRANSMUTE, INTEGRATE, & RENOVATE:
Challenges and Blessings

CHALLENGES FOUND THROUGH RESEARCH	BLESSINGS FOUND THROUGH RESEARCH

MY OWN LIFE EXAMPLES OF THESE CHALLENGES:

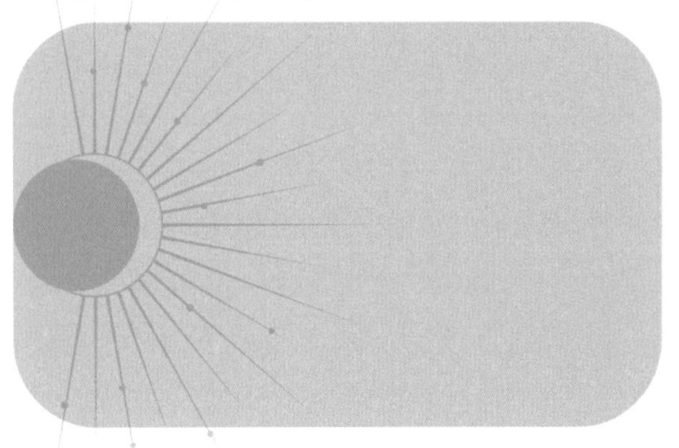

MY OWN LIFE EXPERIENCES OF THESE BLESSINGS:

Lilith

RECLAIMING SOVEREIGNTY

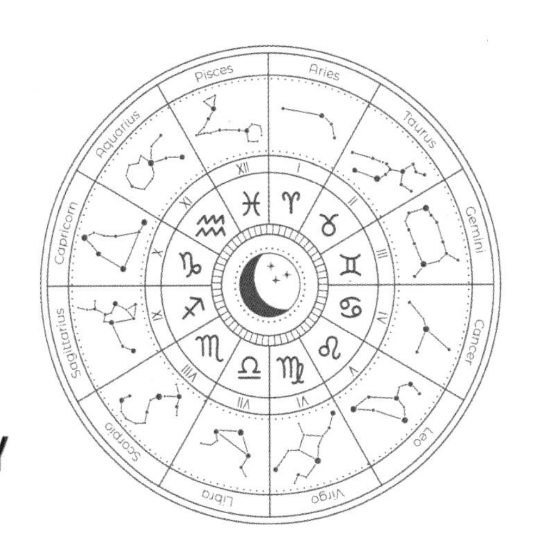

IN WHAT **HOUSE** IS YOUR NATAL LILITH LOCATED?

IN WHAT **SIGN** IS YOUR NATAL LILITH LOCATED?

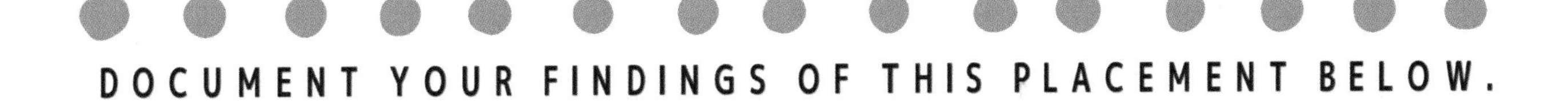

DOCUMENT YOUR FINDINGS OF THIS PLACEMENT BELOW.

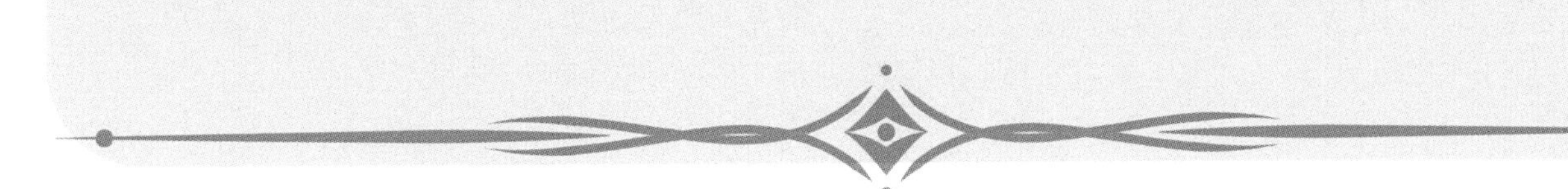

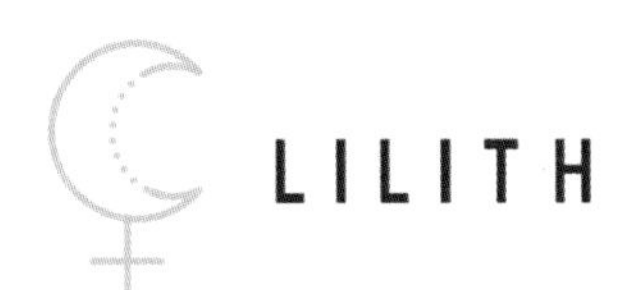

LILITH

Tread with Awareness & Without Judgement.

ALLOW FEELING, SIT IN IT, EXPRESS IT. THROUGH YOUR MOON, LET GO OF RESISTING, LET FEELINGS FLOW THROUGH TO THE SURFACE, TO THE LIGHT.

WRITE & EXPRESS THESE FEELINGS. REPEAT THIS PART AS NEEDED FOR DEEP EMOTIONS TO SETTLE.

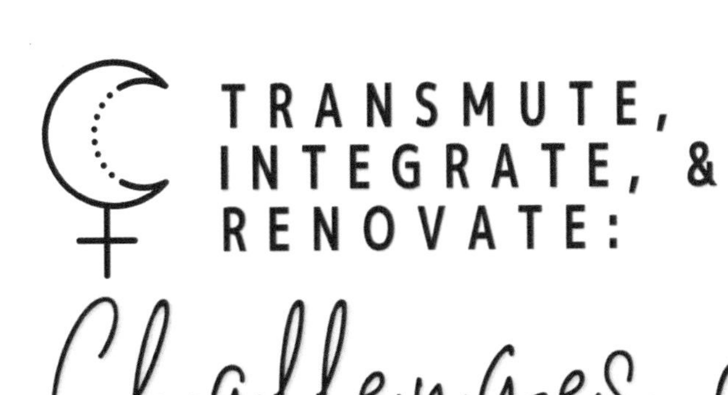

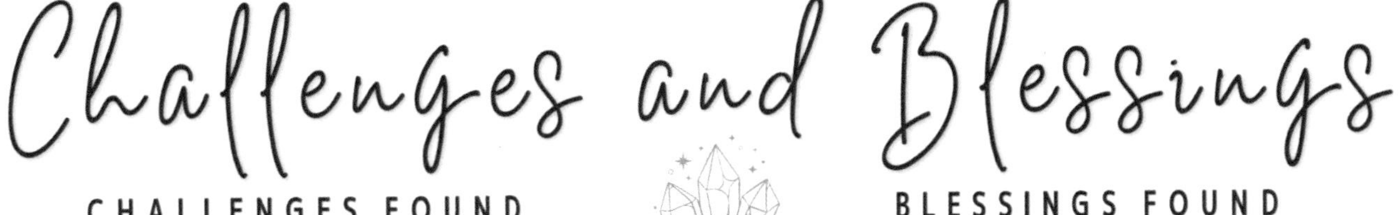

CHALLENGES FOUND THROUGH RESEARCH	BLESSINGS FOUND THROUGH RESEARCH

MY OWN LIFE EXAMPLES OF THESE CHALLENGES:

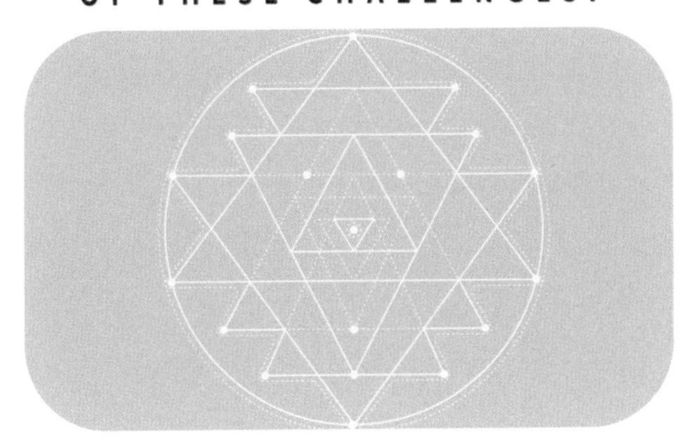

MY OWN LIFE EXPERIENCES OF THESE BLESSINGS:

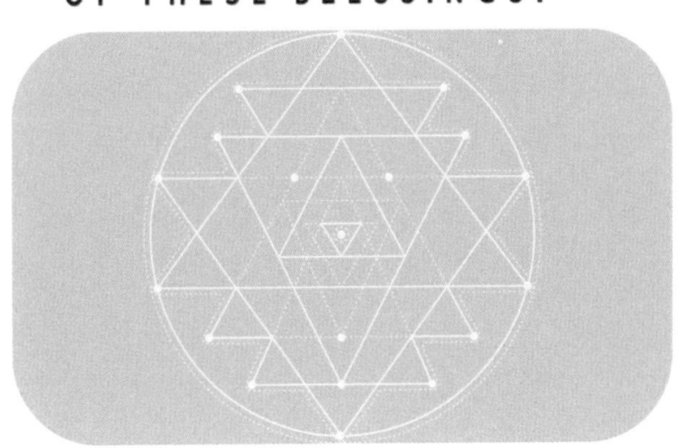

CHIRON

SENSITIVITY INTO STRENGTH

IN WHAT **HOUSE** IS YOUR NATAL CHIRON LOCATED?

IN WHAT **SIGN** IS YOUR NATAL CHIRON LOCATED?

DOCUMENT YOUR FINDINGS OF THIS PLACEMENT BELOW.

CHIRON

Tread with Awareness & Without Judgement.

ALLOW FEELING, SIT IN IT, EXPRESS IT. THROUGH YOUR MOON, LET GO OF RESISTING, LET FEELINGS FLOW THROUGH TO THE SURFACE, TO THE LIGHT.

WRITE & EXPRESS THESE FEELINGS. REPEAT THIS PART AS NEEDED FOR DEEP EMOTIONS TO SETTLE.

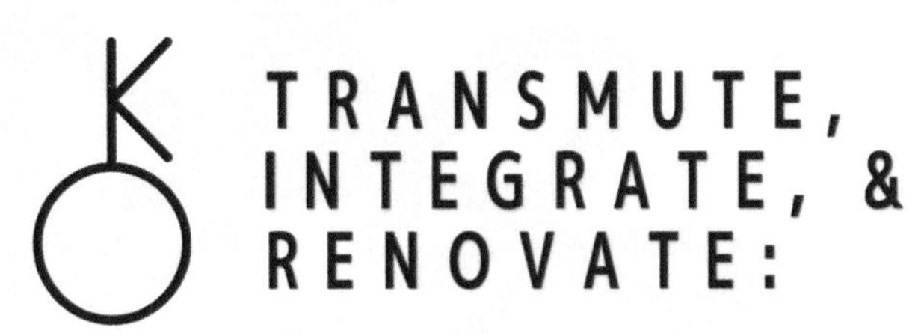

Challenges and Blessings

CHALLENGES FOUND THROUGH RESEARCH	BLESSINGS FOUND THROUGH RESEARCH

MY OWN LIFE EXAMPLES OF THESE CHALLENGES:

MY OWN LIFE EXPERIENCES OF THESE BLESSINGS:

SATURN

REAPING WHAT YOU SOW

IN WHAT **HOUSE** IS YOUR NATAL **SATURN** LOCATED?

IN WHAT **SIGN** IS YOUR NATAL SATURN LOCATED?

DOCUMENT YOUR FINDINGS OF THIS PLACEMENT BELOW.

♄ SATURN

Tread with Awareness & Without Judgement.

ALLOW FEELING, SIT IN IT, EXPRESS IT. THROUGH YOUR MOON, LET GO OF RESISTING, LET FEELINGS FLOW THROUGH TO THE SURFACE, TO THE LIGHT.

WRITE & EXPRESS THESE FEELINGS. REPEAT THIS PART AS NEEDED FOR DEEP EMOTIONS TO SETTLE.

♄ TRANSMUTE, INTEGRATE, & RENOVATE:

Challenges and Blessings

CHALLENGES FOUND THROUGH RESEARCH

BLESSINGS FOUND THROUGH RESEARCH

MY OWN LIFE EXAMPLES OF THESE CHALLENGES:

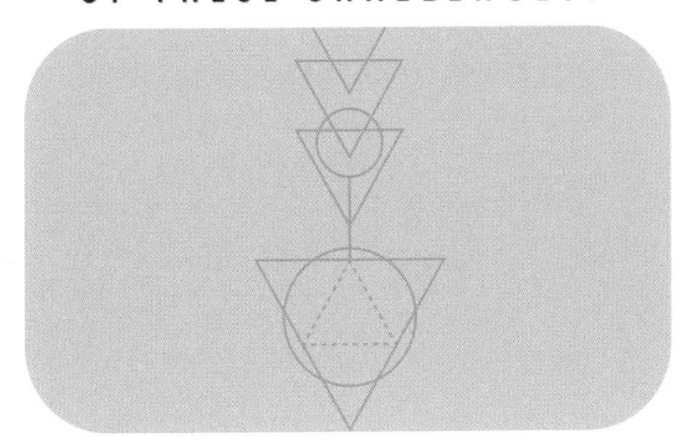

MY OWN LIFE EXPERIENCES OF THESE BLESSINGS:

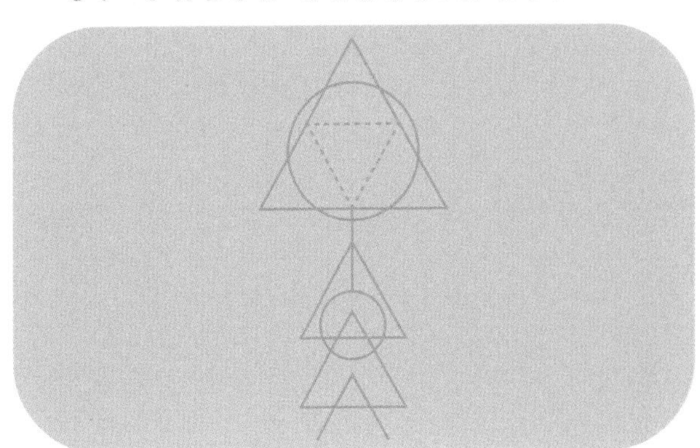

Neptune

DISSOLVING FALSEHOODS

IN WHAT **HOUSE** IS YOUR NATAL NEPTUNE LOCATED?

IN WHAT **SIGN** IS YOUR NATAL NEPTUNE LOCATED?

DOCUMENT YOUR FINDINGS OF THIS PLACEMENT BELOW.

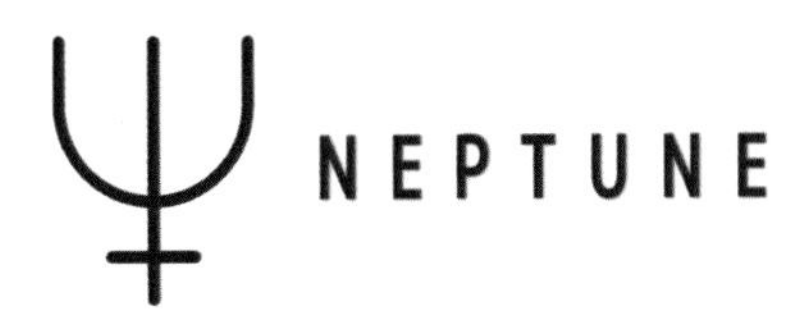

NEPTUNE

Tread with Awareness & Without Judgement.

ALLOW FEELING, SIT IN IT, EXPRESS IT. THROUGH YOUR MOON, LET GO OF RESISTING, LET FEELINGS FLOW THROUGH TO THE SURFACE, TO THE LIGHT.

WRITE & EXPRESS THESE FEELINGS. REPEAT THIS PART AS NEEDED FOR DEEP EMOTIONS TO SETTLE.

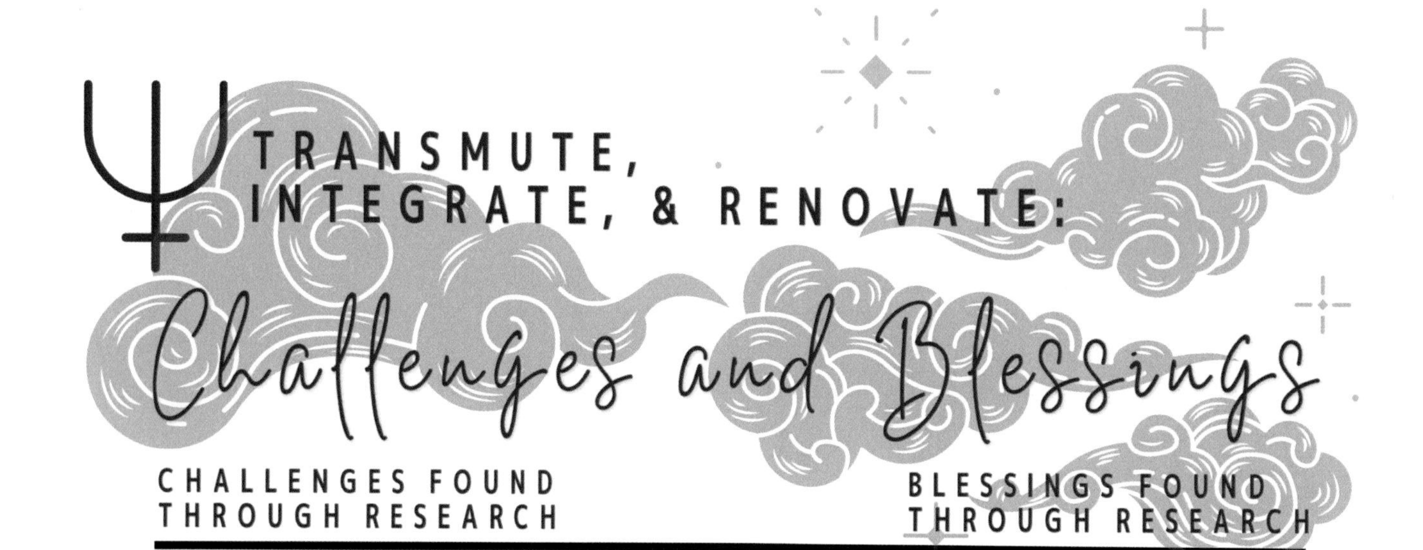

TRANSMUTE, INTEGRATE, & RENOVATE:

Challenges and Blessings

CHALLENGES FOUND THROUGH RESEARCH	BLESSINGS FOUND THROUGH RESEARCH

MY OWN LIFE EXAMPLES OF THESE CHALLENGES:

MY OWN LIFE EXPERIENCES OF THESE BLESSINGS:

Pluto
RISING FROM THE ASHES

IN WHAT **HOUSE** IS YOUR NATAL **PLUTO** LOCATED?

IN WHAT **SIGN** IS YOUR NATAL PLUTO LOCATED?

DOCUMENT YOUR FINDINGS OF THIS PLACEMENT BELOW.

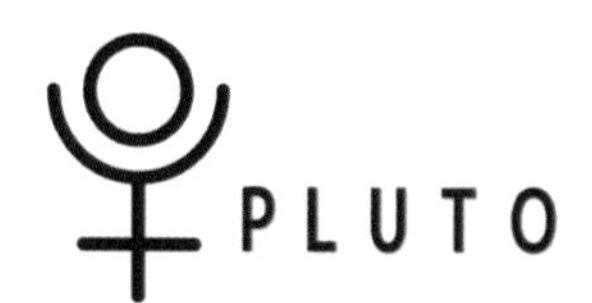

PLUTO

Tread with Awareness & Without Judgement.

ALLOW FEELING, SIT IN IT, EXPRESS IT. THROUGH YOUR MOON, LET GO OF RESISTING, LET FEELINGS FLOW THROUGH TO THE SURFACE, TO THE LIGHT.

WRITE & EXPRESS THESE FEELINGS. REPEAT THIS PART AS NEEDED FOR DEEP EMOTIONS TO SETTLE.

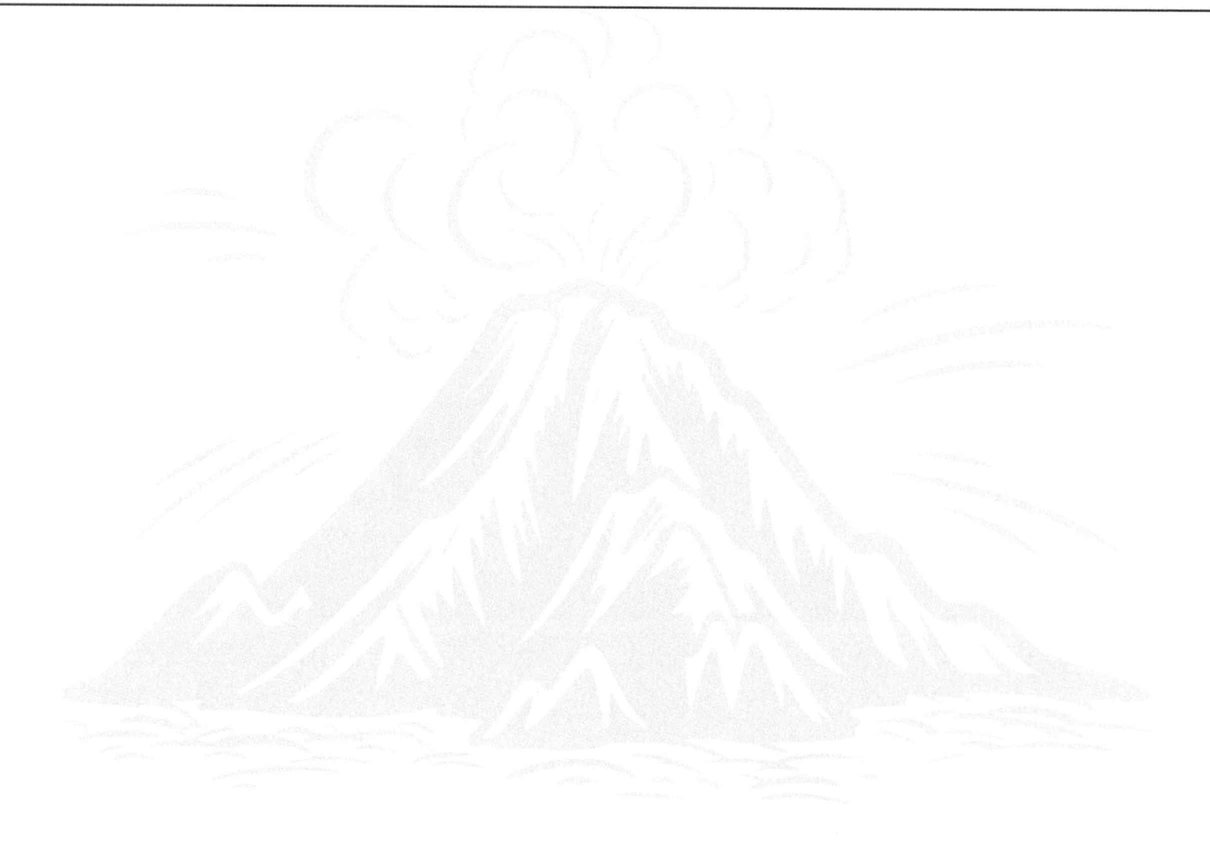

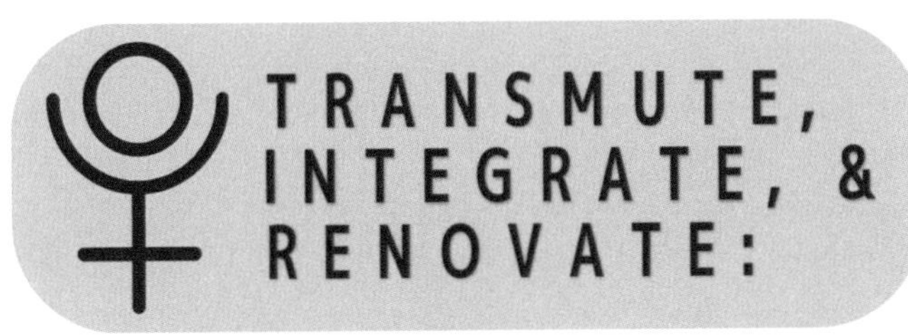

Challenges and Blessings

CHALLENGES FOUND THROUGH RESEARCH	BLESSINGS FOUND THROUGH RESEARCH

MY OWN LIFE EXAMPLES OF THESE CHALLENGES:

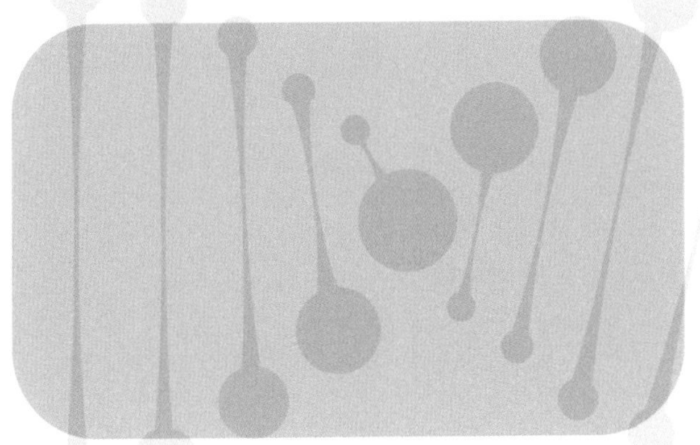

MY OWN LIFE EXPERIENCES OF THESE BLESSINGS:

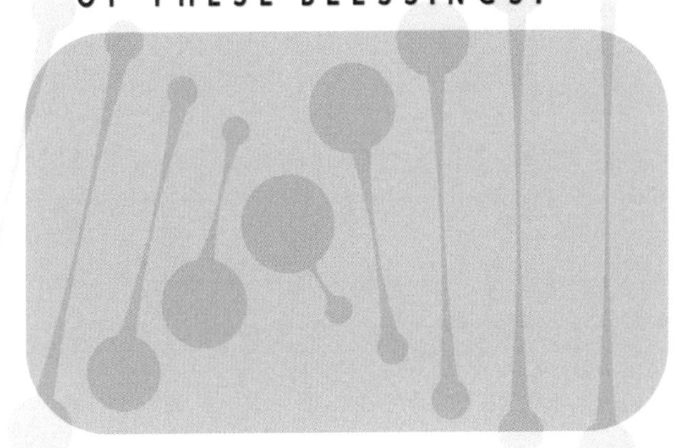

Acknowledgments

These parts...
They guide us.
These challenges...
They strengthen us.
These blessings...
They empower us.

I am grateful to Derrick Naputi and Maggie Kitch for their technical expertise and visual insight. With their open-hearted support, this dream has become even more beautiful than I had imagined.

I am grateful to each and every soul that I have had the blessed opportunity to meet. Many of whom have been patient with my curiosities and questions.

I am grateful to my friends, family, and ancestors who give me life and guidance.

CLOSING REMARKS

I HOPE THIS PROCESS HELPS YOU ALONG YOUR JOURNEY ...

FOR MORE INFORMATION:

EMAIL: MTRAN@2013.NHI.EDU

INSTAGRAM: INSTAGRAM.COM/KHENT84

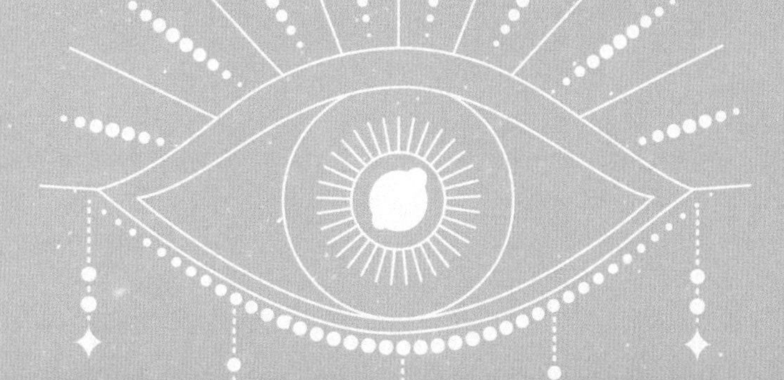

Printed in the United States
by Baker & Taylor Publisher Services